DRAINAGE IN HOMOEOPATHY

DRAINAGE IN HOMOEOPATHY

(DETOXICATION)

by Dr. E. A. MAURY

Translated from the French
by
MARK CLEMENT

THE C. W. DANIEL COMPANY LTD
1 CHURCH PATH, SAFFRON WALDEN,
ESSEX, ENGLAND

2nd Impression December 1982
3rd Impression January 1995

4

ISBN 978 0 850 32069 5

www.randomhouse.co.uk

Penguin Random House is committed to a sustainable future for
our business, our readers and our planet. This book is made from
Forest Stewardship Council® certified paper.

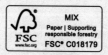

Printed and bound in Great Britain by Clays Ltd, St Ives plc

CONTENTS

INTRODUCTION

During recent years Homoeopathy has taken a preponderant place, especially on the Continent, in the treatment of both acute and chronic affections, and it must necessarily follow the progress of new ideas in Medicine and adapt its practical applications to the modern conception of therapeutics. It is an essential condition of its growing expansion in professional circles as well as among the general public.

It seems clear that Homoeopathy, being an admirable therapeutic method, and having accumulated, since the beginning of the last century, thousands of clinical observations together with an impressive number of cures, must inevitably benefit from any advance made in modern medicine by transcending its own limits when the occasion arises.

This is not to say that we intend to question the validity of the fundamental principle of the method constituting in itself an unalterable foundation on which the whole structure of homoeo-therapeutics is based. A short theoretical and practical account of Homoeopathy was duly given in our *Concise Guide to Homoeopathy* to which the reader is referred.

It is precisely because Homoeopathic Medicine rests on established foundations that it is possible to add another storey, so to speak, to its edifice without running the risk of making it topple down.

There is no question either of modifying in any way the "canon" of the homoeopathic medicinal prescription, based as it is on the law of similars. But it would seem that the time has come when, owing to a new accession of biological and clinical knowledge during the past few decades, a process of "rejuvenation", as it were, should be applied to homoeopathic treatment, as originally conceived by Hahnemann, by introducing a new principle of treatment defined by Dr. Leon Vannier, the eminent leader of the French Homoeopathic School, by the term of "drainage", that is to say detoxication.

The present work, intended for all those practising Homoeopathy in Great Britain and in America, aims at familiarising them with this new principle which has become classical in the teaching and practice of Homoeopathy on the Continent and whose logical application is set out in the following pages.

In order to facilitate the study and understanding of the factors involved, a series of questions, each depending upon the other, has been introduced into each chapter so that the reader may refer to them whenever he feels the need of knowing the answer to any particular question which may occur to him in connection with the theory and practice of "drainage".

8

It is not our aim to discuss biological problems and questions of a physio-pathological nature. While addressing ourselves to doctors in our capacity of homoeopathic physician, we have endeavoured, as far as possible, to make the study of Homoeopathy intelligible to young practitioners as well as to laymen so that the latter, having acquired a clear understanding of the principles involved, may create a favourable atmosphere in which this essentially "human medicine" may thrive, to use the well-known expression coined by Dr. Leon Vannier.

Finally, for the special benefit of practitioners, we have given a condensed *MATERIA MEDICA* of Homoeopathic remedies commonly prescribed in the complementary treatment of "drainage" fully discussed in these pages.

Before repainting a house, the first thing to do is to remove all signs of dirt and dust which have accumulated since it was previously cleaned. In order to obtain a satisfactory result, pleasing and clean, the walls are first washed and the floors swept, and all corners which the broom does not usually reach receive attention so that finally all the dust and debris collected are deposited in the dustbin, generally situated outside the house, on the threshold of the kitchen. It is only when this has been done that the application of fresh coats of paint begins and the renovation process proceeds. The attempt of repainting a house in a dirty and dusty condition may give an illusion of cleanliness but the work is bound to be unsatisfactory for it is only half done.

This analogy, better than long explanations, gives a fairly accurate idea of what homoeopathic "drainage" is pathic remedies indicated according to the law of similars in relation to the sick organism. In brief, it is an organic cleansing process brought about by means of homoeo- and preparing the ground for the more effective action of constitutional remedies.

The conception of "drainage" (detoxication) is as old as that of treatment itself. In ancient medicine it was applied in the form of herbal infusions whose use has been perpetuated until the present time. Artificial sweating, too, represents another modality of organic cleansing which has a certain vogue in the form of steam baths. This conception is not foreign to orthodox medi- cine which uses certain remedies, such as Digitalis, for example, for their diuretic action with a view to "drain- ing" the kidneys.

But these applications of the principle of "drainage" are but partial and relatively limited. Homoeopathy, de- spite its weak influence in orthodox circles, is the Medi- cine of the future, and we are indebted to Dr. Leon Vannier, following Nebel, who, as far back as 1912, began to teach the doctrine of "organic cleansing" as being indispensable to any well-conceived homoeopathic treatment.

As we have already pointed out, while Homoeopathic Medicine remains strictly faithful to the principles laid down by its famous founder, Hahnemann, it must never- theless "rejuvenate" itself, and only in doing so will it be capable of influencing the rising generation of young doctors, on condition, however, that they are given a working instrument that is up to date and adapted to modern scientific ideas.

The present work has been written to fulfil this purpose which is the logical completion of our other works *Concise Guide to Homoeopathy* and *Homoeopathy in 25 Remedies*.

CHAPTER I

WHAT IS "DRAINAGE"?

In the course of this chapter dealing with the therapeutic justification of the complementary method of Homoeopathic "drainage" we propose answering three main questions arising out of the subject matter constituting the present work.

    I.   Definition of "Drainage"

    II. What is meant by Toxins?

    III. How do Toxins act?

I. DEFINITION OF "DRAINAGE"

The general term of "Drainage", that is to say Detoxication, covers the sum total of therapeutic means available to ensure elimination, through natural channels, of toxins vitiating the organism of a patient requiring treatment.

"Drainage" has the dual rôle of performing organic stimulation and elimination of toxins.

An example of "drainage" has already been given in the Introduction in connection with the treatment of fevers by means of herbal infusions, or the application of steam baths in obese arthritic subjects with a view to inducing artificial perspiration, both constituting means of detoxication intended to rid the organism of residual toxins vitiating it periodically.

The body, like an engine, must be cleaned from time to time. This operation may be effected, either spontaneously through the morbid crisis occurring in the course of an affection, and representing, in the last analysis, an effort on the part of the organism to rid itself of its toxins; or by assisting the organism by means of appropriate "drainage" which is the aim of any well-ordered treatment.

In homoeopathic medicine, the means to ensure the natural "drainage" of the patient is provided by the homoeopathic remedies themselves which, when prescribed according to the law of similars, assist the elimination of organic toxins through natural channels. Furthermore, the natural homoeopathic "drainage" fulfils another purpose by preparing the organism for the action of high potencies and safeguarding it against temporary aggravation crises, due to the effects of the remedies administered, and constituting in themselves a manifestation of the drainage process.

II. WHAT IS MEANT BY TOXINS?

This term, somewhat vague in the general sense in which it is employed here, conveniently covers all the various forms of vitiation or infection, and may be understood as representing the different elements of intoxication susceptible of affecting an organism.

For the sake of simplification one may classify the various sources of organic intoxication under three different categories, distinct from one another, but whose manifestations may be found simultaneously in the same subject.

1. Exogenous Toxins—That is to say those which are "external" to the subject, whether they are artificial stimulants, such as alcohol, tobacco, coffee, medicines taken in large doses, or depressing influences, such as worry, anxiety, mental shocks, etc. All these factors, chemical or psychological, act on the tissues of the organism, lowering its resistance and vitiating it.

2. Endogenous Toxins—That is to say those actually found in the subject himself, by which is meant the microbial viruses and toxins associated with tuberculosis, syphilis or any other disease due to microbes and affecting the normal functions of the various systems and organs of the body.

3. Autogenous Toxins—That is to say those generated by the subject himself as a result of his constitution and temperament and transmitted to him through heredity. They affect the organism by lowering its resistance. Arthritism, described by Hahnemann under the term of "Psora", is one of the best examples of this kind of toxins.

From a clinical point of view, there is not a single subject in our modern world who has not been subjected to the effects, either temporary or permanent, of one or the other of these toxins. In other words, it is clear that every patient, before being treated for any affection, must first be "cleansed" in order that the homoeopathic remedy may act with the maximum of efficacy while avoiding, as far as possible, the aggravation crises which may accompany any particular treatment.

III. HOW DO TOXINS ACT?

Whether it is a question of slow-acting toxins, such as alcohol or tobacco; microbial viruses or disorders due to excess of uric acid or oxalic acid, to mention only two end-products of metabolism, the process of intoxication remains the same in all cases.

The first stage consists in progressive vitiation of the organism due to dysfunction of certain organs regulating elimination in different parts of the body.

In the case of alcoholic intoxication the subject presents symptoms of hepatic trouble for the liver cells affected by the toxin of alcohol are no longer able to perform their normal functions. Hence the subject suffers from digestive trouble, lack of appetite, vomiting, to which are added nervous and psychological reactions, all being manifestations of defective functional activity of the liver.

What applies to the liver is equally applicable not only to other organs involved in metabolism, that is to say organs whose function it is to burn up ingested material to render it assimilable by the organism, but also to various endocrine glands, a subject which will be dealt with fully in a subsequent chapter. In our opinion, hormonotherapy in homoeopathic doses, seems to belong to the general conception of "drainage", as it should be understood.

The second stage in the process of intoxication occurs if the practitioner does not intervene in time, or if the patient has no treatment, and consists in the manifestation of a lesion affecting the tissue or organ which has previously been in a state of dysfunction. Disease invariably affects any organ showing the least resistance.

To return to the example already given concerning alcoholic intoxication affecting the liver cells, the lesion which the subject will tend to suffer from consists in sclerosis of the liver together with atrophy of the organ and the pathological consequences resulting from these lesions.

The same applies to other causes of intoxication, whether of microbic or metabolic origin. Thus an excess of uric acid in the blood, being an autogenous toxin, may lead to fixation of the joints causing lesions typical of arthritis or osteo-arthritis.

Medical literature teems with similar examples. Any text-book of clinical pathology, giving a description of various diseases, makes it quite clear that the underlying cause of each one of them is due to an intoxication or infection in the broadest sense of the terms, resulting from the outset in the dysfunction of the organs involved.

Having dealt with these three main questions raised in this chapter, we have established the fact that the application of drainage is absolutely essential in modern

Homoeopathic treatment and should be directed at not only the obvious and temporary cause of the affection but at the whole organism of the patient, including glands and excretory organs.

This process of "organic cleansing" is all the more indispensable as a particular remedy is clearly indicated so that it may act more deeply and with greater efficacy.

CHAPTER II

REASONS FOR "DRAINAGE"

In the course of the preceding chapter we have discussed the general conception of drainage which, in our opinion, is indispensable to any up to date form of homoeopathic treatment. We indicated the aims involved in prescribing drainage remedies, that is to say the fight against organic intoxication.

This conception, giving as it does the key to the complementary therapeutic application, as set out in these pages, must be developed more fully with a view to justifying its unorthodox character to practitioners adhering strictly to the original doctrine of Hahnemann. But everything is bound to evolve. Homoeopathy cannot remain petrified but most broaden its outlook so as to attract more adepts and patients.

In the course of this chapter we propose answering three questions representing a fuller development of the answer to the second question of the preceding chapter.

I. What are the sources of intoxication?

II. Which organs are affected?

III. What benefits are derived from drainage?

I. WHAT ARE THE SOURCES OF INTOXICATION?

When a practitioner who is a homoeopath is confronted by a patient, his first task, after clinical examination which must never be neglected, is to detect the greatest possible number of pathogenetic signs with a view to determining a remedy having the closest "similarity" to them. But he cannot help thinking that his patient in no way resembles the patient of a century ago when Homoeopathy was first put into practice. When referring to the clinical cases given by Hahnemann and his successors it becomes clear that the symptoms described in the course of clinical observation are relatively well defined and that this very clearness leads to a fairly accurate determination of the remedy indicated by the sum total of the signs observed.

At the present time the patient usually comes to the practitioner with a much more complex symptomatology and the pathogenetic signs which, at the time of Hahnemann, were clearly evident and quickly put the physician on the track of the most suitable remedy, have become far less marked in our own time.

We speak from a personal experience extending over a period of 20 years and we must admit that we have to contend with certain difficulties in finding the "similimum".

Why should this be? Because modern man is a deeply intoxicated subject and the variety of causes of organic vitiation confuse the issue and obscure the pathogenetic picture essential for prescribing an efficacious remedy.

Clinical and therapeutic experience have proved that if the sick organism is first cleansed or "drained", the pathogenetic picture will become much clearer and the the determination of the remedy will be rendered easier while its action will be more rapid and effective for the organic reaction resulting from its administration will not be impeded.

In order to prescribe the drainage remedy in accordance with homoeopathic principles it is first necessary to find out the causes of intoxication, that is to say discover the primary cause preventing the full efficacy of the therapeutic action.

We must now return to the three main sources of intoxication discussed in the preceding chapter.

1. INTOXICATION OF EXOGENOUS ORIGIN

We have already seen that these causes spring from elements foreign to the subject. We have also seen that these toxic factors could have either a stimulating or depressing effect on the organism and that they were associated with alcohol, coffee, tea, tobacco, and especially medicines taken in strong doses. In this connection we must also bear in mind certain psychological factors.

2. INTOXICATION DUE TO MEDICINES

This is one of the main causes of organic intoxication for nowadays the average man drugs himself indiscriminately and the medicinal intoxication resulting from this practice constitutes the chief form of gradual intoxication of the organism.

Many patients who consult a homoeopathic practitioner for the first time present a somewhat confused pathogenetic picture from which it is possible to detect two elements: first, the element of the affection itself, and second, the element of medicinal intoxication prior to the onset of the trouble, due to taking large doses of proprietary medicines and such like over a variable period of time.

The homoeopathic practitioner is thus confronted with a double pathogenetic picture, one obscuring the other, and the apparent confusion may well cause difficulty in finding the "similimum", that is to say the remedy really indicated.

In this connection it is interesting to observe the rapidity with which domestic animals and young children given homoeopathic treatment respond to remedies prescribed for them. This is simply due to the fact that their organisms, in the majority of cases, are free from medicinal intoxication and that the pathogenetic signs they present are clear. Moreover, in animals, organic dysfunction is less marked than in humans and therefore the homoeopathic remedy is more efficacious.

3. INTOXICATION DUE TO STIMULANTS

Under this heading are included all products whose excessive use ultimately affects the normal functions of certain organs of elimination, such as coffee, tea, tobacco and alcohol, to mention only the chief ones.

Each of these products causing intoxication acts on one or several organs by modifying normal functions and affecting endocrine glands, and giving rise to a clinical picture whose complexity may well puzzle the practitioner. According to the particular organ affected and the pathogenetic signs presented, an appropriate drainage remedy is prescribed. The organism, having first been cleansed after a few days' treatment, the real clinical and pathogenetic picture will become clearer.

We have already given the example of alcoholic intoxication which, affecting as it does both the liver and the spleen, is benefited by the administration of *Quercus spiritus glandium* which is a specific remedy for the spleen and an antidote to alcohol. By its action on the spleen, this medicine may be regarded as a drainage remedy for this gland, having a secondary effect on the liver.

The action of the best remedy for alcoholic intoxication, *Nux vomica*, will be much more effective if the two organs in question function normally.

The same applies to other causes of intoxication and the reader is referred to the Materia Medica at the end of this work for a list of drainage remedies and their indications.

4. INTOXICATION DUE TO DEPRESSANTS

As already pointed out, the causes of intoxication having a depressing effect include psychological shocks, worry, anxiety, upsetting emotions, all factors having a detrimental effect on the nervous system, and consequently responsible for its abnormal functioning.

It is evident that in these cases, remedies such as *Gelsemium*, *Ignatia* and *Argentum Nitricum*, may be indicated according to the symptoms presented by the patient. But when the nervous system is affected, drainage, by acting on the pituitary or the thyroid gland for example, according to the glandular symptomatology presented, will powerfully assist the action of the constitutional remedy.

5. INTOXICATION DUE TO ENDOGENOUS CAUSES

Under this heading are included all organic intoxications due to microbic agents and toxins properly so-called. They are of two kinds: They may be transmitted by heredity or acquired in the course of life. And here we must make a distinction. Microbic intoxication may be artificially transmitted through vaccination or serotherapy, or may be accidentally acquired by contagion.

Microbic intoxication or viruses, more than toxins of exogenous origin, have a profound effect on all tissues and organs. Whether it is a case of tuberculosis or syphilitic infection, one finds signs of dysfunction in excretory organs due to the presence and action of their specific toxins, and it is in such cases, more than in any other form of intoxication, that drainage is indispensable to allow a deeper and more extensive action of the nosodes indicated without running the risk of aggravation which is always possible.

Tuberculin, for example, generally affects the mucous and serous membranes. By prescribing it at the outset for a patient in whom it is clearly indicated, but who has not been previously prepared by an appropriate drainage, one runs the risk of localising the full effect of the organic reaction on those membranes.

Meningeal symptoms, due to the administration of a high potency of Tuberculin, have been reported. A previous drainage, prescribed in accordance with the specific remedies indicated, will prevent the occurrence of such clinical manifestations which may be sometimes alarming if care has not been taken to "prepare" the patient.

The same may be said of all other remedies given in high potencies.

6. INTOXICATION DUE TO AUTOGENOUS CAUSES

Lastly, one of the causes of organic dysfunction may be due to an intoxication resulting from autogenous toxins being by-products of faulty metabolism.

This especially applies to acquired tendencies through heredity denominated by the somewhat vague though extensive term of arthritism (The Psora of Hahnemann).

It is evident that defective renal function, for example, which may be due to a microbic infection, will assume, in an arthritic subject, a particular importance for the kidneys, being the principal excretory organs of metabolic products, will be liable to dysfunction more easily in arthritic subjects than in normal ones. Hence the possibility of urinary sand or renal calculi (stones) following microbic intoxication of the organs in question.

Let us now give a suitable illustration by taking a subject whose pathogenetic signs call for the prescription of *Medorrhinum*. Let us assume that he is affected by a microbic intoxication of gonococcal origin of long duration and that he has inherited a tendency to arthritism. This predisposition manifests itself in him by pain in the lumbar region.

If, in such a subject who is affected at the same time by an arthritic auto-intoxication and an acquired infection, a dose of *Medorrhinum* in high potency is given at the outset, one runs the risk of throwing an excessive strain on the kidneys which may not be able to perform their excretory functions to the full extent for, according to the clinical signs, the presence of urinary calculi must be suspected. It is therefore advisable in such a case to prescribe first *Berberis,* provided this remedy is homoeopathically indicated, in order to assist the kidneys and enable them to eliminate the toxins which will be released by an ultimate dose of *Medorrhinum* in high potency.

This simple example is given to make it clear how important it is to "drain" the kidneys first and open, as it were, the outlet which will enable the organs to perform their normal functions.

In cases of auto-intoxication, what applies to the kidneys, is equally applicable to other excretory organs or glands functioning in harmony with them.

II. WHICH ORGANS ARE AFFECTED?

The organism being a whole, in Hahnemann's conception, but a whole consisting of small parts, each having its own importance, it is essential to take them and their functions into account.

The aim of Homoeopathic Medicine is to act on the whole but details must not be neglected. Drainage may be said to be one of the main details and the small parts represent various organs through which the process of organic cleansing is effected.

These organs may be classified under two categories, but acting one upon the other respectively: The excretory organs and the endocrine glands.

Each of these organs, performing either an excretory function as regards metabolic by-products, or, in the case of endocrine glands, a stimulating function in the direction of normal metabolism, must be considered whenever homoeopathic treatment is given.

EXCRETORY ORGANS

These include tissues and organs whose function, among others, is to assist the elimination of organic toxins.

The skin plays an important part in this connection as shown by the various cutaneous affections which are but a reflection of a deep-seated trouble. Eczema may be the expression of an arthritic intoxication (Psora) or of an infectious reaction. But if the skin is affected one should bear in mind that it may be due primarily to renal dysfunction, and if the cutaneous affection is to be treated properly, the kidneys should also receive attention. *Berberis*, as an example of drainage remedy, apart from renal symptoms, manifests pathogenetic signs for which it is prescribed in cases of eczema.

The same may be said of the part played by mucous membranes, whether of the respiratory or digestive system, and of serious membranes enveloping and protecting certain organs. Mucous membranes, just like the skin, serve as an outlet for metabolic by-products and toxins, as in the case of diarrhoea often following the administration of *Thuja* in high potency. It is therefore necessary to prepare them for their rôle of elimination.

Among the viscera, we have already mentioned the liver, the spleen, the pancreas which, each in their respective functions, contribute to the cleansing process of the organism. In other words, each of the excretory organs requires a different drainage remedy for each reacts in its own particular manner and presents typical pathogenetic signs.

ENDOCRINE GLANDS

We have already referred to the secondary part played by endocrine glands in the process of elimination manifesting itself as functional stimulation due to various hormones on excretory organs.

In the example given above, that of renal insufficiency in an arthritic subject affected by infectious eczema, the renal function may be stimulated and assisted in its work of secretion and excretion, by giving extract of adrenal gland in weak doses, with the result that its secondary effect invigorates the renal tissue called upon to cleanse the organism. It is in this sense that we regard homoeopathic hormonotherapy as being complementary to drainage

It is not within the scope of the present work to discuss more fully the question of glandular treatment representing a new accretion in the therapeutic field offering new possibilities. It is mentioned here only as being worth remembering and belonging to the general conception of drainage. But it must be pointed out that this technique is in full accord with homoeopathic doctrine for the law of similars can find no better application than in the prescription of glandular extracts, provided they are chosen in accordance with the symptoms of deficiency or excess of glandular functions, as presented by the patient.

We will return to this subject when dealing with the practice of drainage in Chapter IV, in which each organ and gland in particular is considered in relation to the remedies most closely corresponding to them.

The aim of this preliminary study is to stress the importance of drainage in connection with the rôle and functional extent of the excretory organs.

III. WHAT BENEFITS ARE DERIVED FROM DRAINAGE?

We may say that they are of three kinds according as to whether they affect the patient, the treatment, or homoeo-therapeutics in general.

BENEFITS FOR THE PATIENT

By the practice of drainage the patient is safeguarded against the medicinal aggravation due to defective elimination of freed toxins which may occur suddenly following the administration of high potencies, even and especially if the remedy prescribed is clearly indicated.

Let us take an example of a patient whose pathogenetic signs call for the prescription of *Sulphur*. The strain of elimination may affect the kidneys. Let us suppose that the patient's blood urea is increased above the normal level which means that his renal elimination is defective. What is going to happen after a dose of *Sulphur* has been given? The probable appearance of signs of grave renal insufficiency for the kidneys cannot cope with the strain imposed on them with the result that drowsiness and depression ensue, in short, a clinical picture causing alarm to the practitioner and anxiety to the patient.

If the precaution had been taken at the outset to assist the kidneys and to reduce the amount of blood urea, the dose of *Sulphur* would have acted without causing those manifestations of aggravation which often make the patient give up homoeopathic treatment. It is the reason for which, and this cannot be sufficiently emphasised, Homoeopathy cannot dispense with clinical examination and laboratory tests as well.

The sequence of events, in the case of the administration of *Sulphur*, may be repeated when other remedies in high potencies are prescribed.

BENEFITS FOR THE TREATMENT

The benefits accruing to the treatment as a result of the application of drainage are manifested by its shorter duration. It would appear that by first treating the excretory organs or the endocrine glands the action of the remedy prescribed is, in some way, activated and enables it to have a more rapid effect.

It seems to us that prescribing the same remedy for months, though clearly indicated, in order to obtain an improvement in the pathological condition, is rather a waste of time. If the patient feels better at the end of a long period of treatment, one may attribute the cure, not to the action of the homoeopathic remedy itself but simply to Nature. It is then difficult to know what really effected the cure.

Drainage, by assisting elimination, assists at the same time the action of the remedy prescribed and hastens the process of cure which may justly be attributed to the homoeopathic remedy itself.

BENEFITS FOR HOMOEOPATHY

The benefits that Homoeopathy may derive from the application of drainage result normally from what has been described above.

If the patient is rapidly cured, without any aggravation, he becomes a convert to the homoeopathic method of treatment for he has experienced its benefits. On the other hand, if the practitioner knows how to treat his patient correctly according to the technique we advocate, he safeguards him against the possibility of medicinal aggravation and understands his condition better, for the pathogenetic symptoms become clearer and improvement occurs more quickly than is the case otherwise. The practitioner becomes convinced therefore of the validity of homoeopathic doctrine and will devote his activities to its expansion.

If Homoeopathy is to thrive, it behoves us to bring about such conditions that both the patient treated and the practitioner not only accept is principles but also become fully aware of the benefits to be derived from their application.

We believe that the drainage method, properly understood and applied in accordance with the principles laid down in the present work, constitutes an appreciable advance in the domain of modern Homoeopathy.

CHAPTER III

HOW "DRAINAGE" ACTS

In the two preceding chapters we have established the fact that the homoeopathic practitioner must necessarily bear in mind that the choice of remedy, especially when given in high potencies, depends on certain factors and pre-supposes a beneficial action, relatively rapid, for contrary to what is generally believed, Homoeopathy in cases where the remedy is indicated in strict accordance with the law of similars, is a method of treatment achieving very rapid results.

For the sake of clearness, the factors involved are summed up below:

1. The remedy must be chosen correctly, that is to say it must have a close "similarity" to the real pathogenetic signs presented by the patient. In order to have an accurate picture of the real affection, that is to say of the sum total of symptoms and signs causing the lesion or dysfunction under consideration, it is first essential to "cleanse" the subject of metabolic by-products or toxins vitiating the organism and often blurring the real clinical picture.

We have already dealt with this point at length.

2. It is also desirable that the remedy should act rapidly, not in the course of a few months, but within a few weeks or days, without giving rise, at the outset of the treatment, to alarming reactions in the form of aggravation of symptoms due to sudden elimination of products or toxins vitiating the organism under treatment. This point has also been dealt with previously.

3. Having established these fundamental facts it becomes clearly evident that the patient must first be treated by means of drainage which reduces the toxic tension in the blood, stimulates the action of the cells and assists the free elimination of toxins, whatever their nature may be.

4. Lastly, the process of toxin elimination is effected through tissues such as the skin and mucous membranes, as well as through certain viscera having an excretory function such as the liver, kidneys and pancreas.

With regard to the process of stimulating cellular activity, this is mediated through the endocrine glands, some of which are acting on the blood (spleen) while others, having more complex functions, may be regarded as adjuvants to drainage (adrenal, pituitary, thyroid, sexual glands).

We shall refer to these points again in the course of the present chapter.

Having thus established the validity of the technique of drainage it is incumbent upon us to explain how drainage acts, and the formulation of an acceptable hypothesis is called for.

There are three questions which must be dealt with.

1. What is the part played by the excretory organs?

2. What is the part played by the endocrine glands?

3. Why the drainage remedy must be linked up with the constitutional remedy.

1. WHAT IS THE PART PLAYED BY THE EXCRETORY ORGANS?

In the course of the preceding chapter, in connection with the question "Which organs are affected?" the conception of the intervention and action of excretory organs in the treatment of disease was outlined, whether the latter was functional or organic.

Any affection may be regarded, in the last analysis, as a manifestation of defensive reaction on the part of the organism towards toxins accumulating in its tissues. The morbid crisis is an expression of this attempt to rid the body, either suddenly or gradually, of metabolic by-products or excessive toxins. These, under the influence of treatment are excreted through the natural outlets of the organism and are incorporated with the urine, faeces, sweat, bile, digestive juices, and in certain pathological conditions, with pus or fluids resulting from reactive secretions such as effusions.

In other words, the main excretory organs, that is to say organs of elimination, are the skin, the mucous membranes of the respiratory, digestive and genital systems, the viscera (liver, pancreas, kidneys). We must consider the pathological manifestations observed in them as being an expression of an attempt to free the organism from organic toxins.

The function of the practitioner therefore is to assist the organism in this cleansing process through the affected tissues by means of various therapeutic measures at his disposal, and Homoeopathy provides some excellent ones.

Let us again draw attention to the reaction of the skin when it is subjected to an excessive elimination of toxins which, instead of passing through the kidneys, which are not functioning normally, is diverted to the cutaneous surface. The resulting reaction takes the form of eczema being a manifestation of organic intoxication.

We must also consider what takes place in cases in which the kidneys, not functioning normally, and organically affected, are no longer capable of playing their part in the process of elimination.

The patient, especially if he has attained a certain age, shows symptoms of high blood urea whose importance and dangerous reaction have already been pointed out when remedies in high potencies are administered.

With regard to the mucous membranes of the digestive system, the process of elimination may be accompanied by vomiting and diarrhoea calling for appropriate drainage remedies to assist the detoxication of the organism.

Observing the patient with a little common sense should be sufficient to make the practitioner realise the value and significance of the symptoms presented, many of which being due to the effort on the part of the organism of ridding itself of toxins. The symptoms call for an "adjuvant" remedy, that is to say a drainage remedy.

To sum up, we may say that the excretory organs act as "thresholds of elimination" whose integrity must be maintained in view of their important functions.

2. WHAT IS THE PART PLAYED BY ENDOCRINE GLANDS?

We have already discussed this question on several occasions. The complementary part of drainage played by an endocrine gland consists, in our opinion, in communicating the stimulating action necessary to the sum total of the organic functions, including nutrition, reproduction, respiration and circulation.

Any function implies a dual task, one of assimilation and the other of excretion of products resulting from the first process. A burning fire is invariably accompanied by the formation of ashes which must be cleared away from the grate so that the flames may be maintained and the heat allowed to spread as desired. The same applies to the human organism. The ingestion of various materials essential for the maintenance of life (foods, drinks, air, etc.) may be compared to coal burnt in a furnace to keep the fire going. If perfect organic combustion is required it is necessary not only to clean the biological furnace from time to time and remove the accumulated ashes but also to let in sufficient air to keep up the indispensable process of combustion. This is precisely the part played by the endocrine glands with their internal secretions. Thanks to their specific metabolic action on certain excretory organs, their hormones assist the cleansing process by stimulating the tissues whose functions are slowed down, and consequently facilitating indirectly the natural elimination of by-products and toxins whose importance in vitiating the organism has been emphasised already.

It is not our intention to discuss the stimulating action of every endocrine gland in the body in this work. As in our former works, *Concise Guide to Homoeopathy* and *Homoeopathy in 25 Remedies*, the present work aims at being essentially practical. But in order to give a clear understanding of the compensatory and adjuvant action of an endocrine gland we will give an example taken from our personal experience.

In certain cases of arterial hypertension we have often prescribed *Thyroidea* as a drainage remedy in homoeopathic doses, independently of the constitutional remedy indicated by the sum total of symptoms presented by the patient. As a result, there has invariably been a fairly rapid fall of blood pressure. Why should this occur? In many patients, a rise of arterial tension may be regarded as an effort on the part of the organism to rid itself of an excess of urea which vitiates the blood and which may be due to excessive nervous or psychological strain. In such cases, especially if there are also symptoms of tobacco intoxication, a frequent occurrence, the thyroid gland, which is very sensitive to the action of nicotine, is in a state of hyperactivity and the product of its internal secretion increases in varying amounts and affects the tone of the arterial walls by communicating to them the increase of muscular and nervous tension with the result that the arterial pressure rises. Moreover, the metabolic by-products carried by the blood pass through the contracted arterial walls with some difficulty and this further complicates the process of elimination.

Thus by giving *Thyroidea* in homoeopathic doses and in accordance with Hahnemann's doctrine, for we are actually applying the law of similars, the arterial walls will be relaxed and able to allow the free passage of urea in the blood into the kidneys whose function it is to excrete it normally. The latter, in their turn, correctly "drained", will be able to carry out their excretory function, and consequently the amount of urea in the blood will be decreased and the arterial tension lowered, both manifestations of organic cleansing correctly realised.

The example given concerning the action of the thyroid gland is equally applicable to any other endocrine gland when its action is considered from this particular point of view. All that is needed is to understand the relations connecting them together and to consider some of their functions within the framework of what has been discussed in the course of this chapter.

Endocrine glands, therefore, act as compensating and stimulating agents in the process of drainage.

3. WHY DRAINAGE AND CONSTITUTIONAL REMEDIES MUST BE LINKED UP

Two main objections may be raised by homoeopaths accustomed to the discipline of the pure doctrine of Homoeopathy sanctioning, in principle, but a single remedy prescribed in accordance with precise pathogenetic indications at varying intervals. One objection is to deny the efficacy of the technique of drainage, and the other is to regard this complementary treatment as damaging to orthodox Homoeopathy.

It may thus be levelled against us that we may be practising a good system of Medicine but not Homoeopathy. And yet, did not Hahnemann himself, as we may read in the 6th edition of his famous classic work the "Organon", practise drainage to prevent medicinal aggravation when he resorted to a method consisting in giving the chosen remedy by repeating it fairly frequently, sometimes daily, but each time in a different potency, according to an increasing series.

Dr. Tyler, too, administered certain remedies in three successive doses taken during three days and also in increasing potencies.

We have already dealt with the two main objections mentioned in the course of the preceding chapter, and when the question of the practice of drainage is discussed in the next chapter we shall stress the necessity of choosing the drainage remedy in strict accordance with the law constituting the basis of homoeopathic treatment.

Lastly, we think it is necessary to discuss this question once again in order to justify to the fullest extent the application of the technique of drainage.

By carefully chosen examples we have shown why the drainage remedy must necessarily accompany the prescription of the constitutional remedy. The action of the remedy given in high potency gives rise in the organism to a new functional activity affecting the different systems involved in the process of metabolism and stimulating them in a beneficial manner with a view to restoring the patient to health.

The homoeopathic remedy, in our view, plays the rôle of a "catalyst", not only specific in regard to the affection to be treated but also specific in regard to the tissues or organs affected. This process of catalysis, of which we have given a few examples and proofs, is accompanied by the formation of by-products and infectious toxins, and therefore one must anticipate that the organism will react by an elimination crisis generally manifesting itself in the affected organ.

Drainage, directed at the organ in question, prepares it, in some way, to cope with the effects of this beneficial shock, and that is the reason why it must be made adaptable to it.

At the risk of repetition we cannot sufficiently stress this conception which, when thoroughly understood and properly applied, seems to form a logical and essential part of any complete treatment.

The drainage remedy is, therefore, associated with the constitutional remedy because it assists the latter in its action.

CHAPTER IV

HOW TO PRACTISE "DRAINAGE"

Having attempted to make the reader understand the necessity of drainage in the course of homoeopathic treatment and having justified its application, there remains only one question to be discussed, namely, how the technique should be applied.

Let us point out once again that the drainage remedy, being added to or preceding the constitutional remedy, is a remedy having a selective action on the particular tissue or organ whose functioning is disturbed, and which owing to this disturbance, prevents the free elimination of organic by-products and toxins.

The application of drainage is subject to certain rules originating directly from the homoeopathic doctrine as will be seen in the course of the answers given to the following three questions.

I.   How to choose drainage remedies?

II. What are the dangers to avoid?

III. Which are the drainage remedies?

In answering these three questions we have endeavoured to give the essential points concerning the subject. We do not claim to have considered the subject as completely as it should be for there are certain questions, especially in the domain of physio-biology, that might be profitably discussed, but we must bear in mind that the present work aims at being practical and easily comprehensible to the general public.

1. HOW TO CHOOSE DRAINAGE REMEDIES?

At the outset, we must stress the fact that the choice of a drainage remedy is strictly determined by the Materia Medica, that is to say it is entirely dependent on the signs corresponding most closely to the morbid symptoms observed. In other words, the drainage remedy must correspond, by its exact "similarity", to the transient symptoms of the actual state of the affection in progress.

There are three factors involved in determining the choice of a remedy so that the latter may really represent the "similimum" according to the law constituting the basis of Homoeopathy.

(a) THE CLINICAL FACTOR

This is connected with the examination of the patient carried out, not only by means of the usual interrogation characteristic of homoeopathic technique, bearing on the determination of physical signs indicating a certain remedy as well as on psychological signs whose importance in Homoeopathy is considerable, but also by means of clinical examination constituting the customary medical routine whose results may have to be confirmed by laboratory tests and X-ray examinations.

The practitioner will thus be in a position to determine beforehand the particular organ, system or gland which may be affected by the reaction of the organism. Generally speaking, it is the weakest organ or that which is affected by pain or some functional trouble.

The question arises as to which system or tissue will be affected in principle, by the process of organic cleansing in an arthritic. As a rule, in such a case, the patient may show symptoms of eczema (cutaneous localisation) or asthma (bronchial localisation), or lumbar pain (renal localisation). In the latter case, an X-ray examination of the kidneys may be called for which may reveal the presence of a urinary calculus (stone). The practitioner having established his clinical diagnosis will know that since the kidney, an excretory organ, is affected he will have to take the necessary measures to "prepare" it to meet the crisis that will result from the administration of a homoeopathic remedy in high potency. He will thus have to make a choice among the drainage remedies of the renal functions which will lead him to consider the second factor discussed below.

(b) THE HOMOEOPATHIC FACTOR

To retain the example given previously, the practitioner will thus be "clinically" directed towards a trouble of the renal functions.

In consulting the Materia Medica in regard to drainage remedies there are several of them which seem to be indicated in this particular case, notably *Berberis, Chima-*

phila, *Sarsaparilla*, each one having different pathogenetic signs and modalities but all acting equally on the urinary function.

Berberis, for example, is associated with burning pain in the renal region and acute pain during micturition.

Chimaphila has, among its indications, a constant desire to micturate with a sensation of fullness in the perineum.

Sarsaparilla is associated rather with a right renal localisation and unbearable pain at the end of micturition.

It will thus be seen, as pointed out at the outset, how important it is, once the clinical diagnosis has been established, to look carefully in the patient for homoeopathic medicinal signs "similar" to those observed in the affected subject, in order to be able to determine an appropriate therapeutic diagnosis.

In other words, the drainage remedies are not specific for certain affections and are not the same for the same type of affection. They vary according to the cause of the intoxication, even if the morbid localisation occurs in the same system.

We must refer once more to the example of the arthritic (or psoric patient suffering from a renal calculus (stone)) for which *Calcarea carbonica* is indicated as a constitutional remedy.

This patient, whose urinary system must be "drained", may show indications, according to the signs presented, for *Berberis*, as a complementary remedy, if the localisation is clearly renal, or for *Chimaphila*, if the localisation is prostatic, or for *Sarsaparilla* if the localisation is urethral. But in each case, different pathgenetic signs will be observed.

The drainage remedy, therefore, must be homoeopathetically "individualised", and it is precisely this necessity which justifies its administration in accordance with the principles of homoeopathic doctrine.

(c) THE COMPLEMENTARY FACTOR

This is the last factor we have to consider in connection with the choice of the drainage remedy. The latter must be, in effect, adapted to the constitutional remedy. It must be, in some way, "complementary", that is to say that its particular action on a certain organ must assist the general action of the constitutional remedy.

Taking the example of a patient for whom *Lycopodium* is indicated with the object of treating a condition of auto-intoxication of hepatic origin, certain pathogenetic signs observed in the patient will lead to the prescription of *Solidago*, as a drainage remedy, which has in its pathogenesis signs of hepatic insufficiency with faulty metabolism of protein by-products. The complementary action of this remedy will assist the constitutional action of *Lycopodium* and ensure a thorough cleansing process of the organism.

II. WHAT ARE THE DANGERS TO AVOID?

In principle, there are three main dangers which must be briefly discussed.

(a) MECHANICAL PRESCRIBING

Owing to the necessity of giving a drainage remedy that is both individualised and homoeopathically indicated by the signs observed, mechanical prescribing is thus avoided, that is to say the practitioner will not prescribe blindly any particular remedy without having first established a homoeopathic diagnosis.

(b) ABUSE OR PROLONGED ADMINISTRATION OF LOW POTENCIES

This danger assumes a certain importance owing to the fact that the continued administration of a drainage remedy, approximating in strength to the mother tincture, may give rise in the patient to a real pathogenesis whose symptoms represent the reaction of the organism towards the remedy which is abused. There is a risk, in such a case, of bringing about a real medicinal intoxication mentioned at the beginning of the present work.

The drainage remedy would thus have an effect contrary to that it is intended to have.

(c) Lastly, one must avoid giving complex prescriptions in which the practitioner, in order to cope with all possibilities, prescribes several associated drainage remedies. A single drainage remedy should suffice, the reason for this having already been given, provided it is prescribed according to the pathogentic symptoms observed.

In a case of complex drainage it would be difficult to know which remedy had been really efficacious if, by any chance, an improvement resulted.

It is possible to lay down the following rule: A single homoeopathic remedy, a single drainage remedy but individualised and homoeopathically indicated.

III. WHICH ARE THE DRAINAGE REMEDIES?

The answer to this question which is the last we have to consider to complete our summary exposition of the technique of drainage will enable us to give a list of remedies whose classification will be established according to their particular mode of action. But before proceeding to do so, we must point out that, according to the principle discussed in the preceding chapter, any homoeopathic remedy given in low potency (1x or 3x) may be regarded as a drainage remedy.

The list of remedies given here and briefly discussed in the next chapter on Materia Medica have been specially selected because they have a particularly specific action on the affected organ, system or tissue whose functional activity is defective.

We may thus divide drainage remedies into three categories, the organo-therapeutic remedies, the remedies adapted to constitutional remedies and the hormono-therapeutic remedies. But we repeat that they must be prescribed in accordance with precise pathogenetic indications which will be referred to again in the Materia Medica.

With regard to dosage, they should be given once or twice a day, in the form of one or two pilules, or 5 drops before meals.

1. ORGANO-THERAPEUTIC REMEDIES

These are drainage remedies having a selective action on certain tissues or organs. They must be classified as follows:

Action on the

Skin: Calendula, Cyrtopodium, Petroleum.

Mucous Membranes: Hydrastis, Sedum acre.

Nervous System: Arnica, Gelsemium, Ignatia.

Digestive System:

Stomach: Condurango, Ornithogallum.

Rectum: Hura Braz, Ruta, Scrofularia.

Liver: Carduus mar, Chelidonium, Cinchona, Conium, Taraxacum, Solidago.

Pancreas: Senna.

Urinary System:

Kidneys: Berberis, Formica rufa, Sarsaparilla, Solidago.

Prostate: Chimaphila.

Uterus: Helonias, Thlaspi Bursa past.

REMEDIES ADAPTED TO CONSTITUTIONAL REMEDIES

We have already discussed the question of the concomitant prescription of these drainage remedies with those given in high potencies. This is stressed again here.

Besides the great polycrests having a deep action on the subject in whom it is indicated by his pathogenetic signs, like *Natrum mur, Sulphur, Sepia, Lycopodium,* etc., there are "families of remedies" whose action reinforces or is complementary to the effect of polycrest and which are prescribed, particularly in acute cases, for patients in whom they are indicated.

For example, one may think of giving as a drainage remedy to a patient for whom *Natrum mur* is indicated as a constitutional remedy in an acute case, such remedies as *Apis, Abrotanum, Pulsatilla.*

These special drainage remedies may also be divided into several categories according to their specific action.

Action on Infections:
> **Tuberculosis:** Crataegus, Pulsatilla, Rhus tox.
> **Syphilis:** Aurum, Phytolacca, Platina, Plumbum.

Action on **Diabetes:** Argentum nitricum, Conium, Helonias, Hydrastis.

HORMONOTHERAPEUTIC REMEDIES

As already pointed out, these drainage remedies have a specific action on endocrine glands. Apart from remedies extracted from the glands themselves, such as *Thyroidea*, for example, which are as varied as the glands or hormones themselves, there are a number of drainage remedies derived from the vegetable kingdom, which have a specific action on certain glands of the organism.

Spleen: Ceanothus, Quercus spiritus glandium.

Mammary gland: Asterias rubens, Phytolacca, Scrofularia.

We shall discuss each of these drainage remedies in the chapter on Materia Medica but we advise the practitioner who may be called upon to prescribe them, according to the principles laid down in the present work, to consult first a standard text-book of Homoeopathic Materia Medica in order that he may obtain a more thorough knowledge of them and be able to check up the pathogenetic signs corresponding to those observed in the patient.

CONCLUSIONS

Our aim in this little manual has been to give the essential characteristics of what must be understood under the general term of "Drainage".

Any organism undergoing an acute crisis or presenting a chronic pathological condition must be freed from by-products of metabolism or elements of intoxication preventing the normal functions of the organs.

This cleansing process, set into action by a homoeopathic remedy given in high potency, must first be prepared or assisted by the action of drainage remedies on the excretory organs and endocrine glands. The drainage remedy must be chosen according to the pathogenetic signs observed in the patient to be treated and given in low potency, once or twice a day in the course of the administration of the constitutional remedy.

Thus the dangers of medicinal aggravation will be avoided and the cure of the patient speeded up.

These are the two aims which the homoeopathic practitioner must constantly bear in mind for the welfare of his patient.

CHAPTER V

MATERIA MEDICA

Within the scope of the present work we can give only a selection of drainage remedies chosen from those which are considered most important and are most frequently indicated, and characterise each one by brief symptomatological notes.

We strongly advise that they should be prescribed, not only according to their clinical indications but also and particularly according to their indications of similarity to the signs observed in the patient under treatment.

As this subject is fully treated in the standard textbooks of Homoeopathic Materia Medica, we have confined ourselves to giving only the leading symptoms and indications which must be supplemented by consulting the major works.

Argentum Nit.

Action on certain diatheses (constitutional dispositions).
Nervous system deeply affected; phobias, apprehension, depression.
Weakness with tremors; giddiness.
Irritation of mucous membranes.

Arnica

Action on the nervous system.
Deep depression, physical and mental; intense fatigue; insomnia.
Nervous exhaustion.

Asterias rub.

Action on mammary glands.
Congestion of left breast and pain; induration of breast; sub-axillary adenopathy.

Aurum

Action on syphilitic subjects.
Induration and hypertrophy of congested organs.
Tendency to suicide. Pains in bones.

Berberis

Action on the kidneys.
Rheumatic diathesis; renal colic with burning sensation in kidney region; scalding pain during micturition.

Calendula

Action on the skin.
Activates healing of wounds; prevents suppuration and ulceration.

Carduus mur.

Action on the liver.

Congestion of liver with hepatic dysfunction; tendency to haemorrhage; pain in right side; nausea, bitter taste in mouth; yellow skin.

Ceanothus

Action on the spleen.

Deep pain in left hypochondrium; splenomegaly.

Chelidonium

Action on the liver.

Constant pain in liver and inferior angle of right scapula; sub-icterus of conjunctiva.

Pultaceous and yellowish stools; dark urine.

Chimaphila

Action on the prostate.

Genito-urinary troubles.

Constant desire to micturate; sensation of heaviness in perineum.

Cinchona off.

Action on the liver.

Bitter taste in mouth; abdominal distension.

Yellowish diarrhoea, after meals.

Liver enlarged and tender.

Condurango

Action on the stomach.

Cancerous infiltration of gastric mucosa.

Burning pains in stomach.

Conium

Action on the liver, mammary glands and certain diatheses.
Induration of glands; indurated lumps in breasts.
Abdomen, hard and tense; hepatic pains.
Ascending paralysis.

Crataegus

Action on tuberculous subjects.
Cardiac fatigue on least exercise; weak pulse, rapid and irregular.

Cyrtopodium

Action on the skin.
Accelerates healing of furuncles.

Formica rufa

Action on the kidneys.
Urinary troubles with rheumatic diathesis.
Urine, abundant and turbid, at night.

Gelsemium

Action on the nervous system.
Physical and mental weakness with tremors.
Harmful effects of emotional or psychological shocks.

Helonias

Action on the uterus.
Uterine prolapse.
Pain in dorso-lumbar region; patient is "uterus conscious".

Hura Braz.

Action on the rectum.
Intense burning pains in anus with sensation of constriction.
Constipation with ineffective desire; haemorrhoids.

Hydrastis

Action on the mucous membranes and in certain diatheses
Glandular troubles; discharge from mucous membranes, thick and yellowish.
Pre-cancerous states; ulceration.

Ignatia

Action on the nervous system.
Psychological troubles; dysfunction of sympathetic nervous system following emotional shocks; nervous fatigue.
Paradoxical character of symptoms and sensations.
Mental depression; contradictory pains.

Ornithogallum

Action on the stomach.
Pre-cancerous or cancerous state of the mucous membranes.
Pains in the stomach radiating to thorax and legs; acid vomiting.

Petroleum

Action on the skin.
Skin, dry and fissured; chilblains in winter, especially in fingers.
Oozing eruptions, burning and pruriginous vesicles.

Phytolacca

Action on syphilitic subjects, mucous membranes of pharynx, mammary glands and lymphatic glands.
Pains in bones.
Glandular induration.

Platina

Action on syphilitic subjects.
Alternation of physical and psychological symptoms.
Pains of pressure and cramps, appearing and disappearing gradually.

Plumbum

Action on syphilitic subjects.
Loss of weight with physical and mental weakness.
Progressive paralysis of limbs.

Pulsatilla

Action on tuberculous subjects.
Venous congestion of extremities.
Secretions, thick, yellowish and non-irritating.
Tendency to chilliness.

Quercus spiritus Gl.

Action on the spleen.
Pain in left hypochondrium; splenomegaly.

Rhus tox.

Action on tuberculous subjects.
Generalised stiffness.
Pains of infectious origin; restlessness; shivering with dry cough.

Ruta

Action on the rectum.
Stools, blood-stained and difficult to expel.
Cancer of the rectum.

Sarsaparilla

Action on the kidneys.
Intense pain in right kidney; urinary sand.
Intolerable pain at end of micturition.

Scrofularia

Action on the rectum.
Pain in rectum; bleeding and painful haemorrhoids.

Sedum acre

Action on the mucous membranes.
Tendency to fissure, especially in anal mucous membrane.

Senna

Action on the pancreas.
Aromatic odour of breath; acetonaemia in children.

Solidago

Action on the liver and kidneys.
Hepatic and renal insufficiency; pain in costo-vertebral angle in lumbar region.
Abdominal distension; constipation; urine, scanty and dark.

Taraxacum

Action on the liver.
Sub-icterus of conjunctiva; tongue, patchy, white with dark red areas.
Jaundice with hepatic pain.

Thlaspi Bursa past.

Action on the uterus.

Premature periods, abundant with black coagulated blood.

Metrorrhagia (Bleeding from the womb apart from proper periods).